<u>Emotional Eating - Myth vs Reality</u>

The What? The Why?

and Solutions of Emotional Eating

By Dunstamac

The aim of this book is to provide true and credible details on the issue at hand. The publisher is not obliged to offer accounting, lawfully approved, or otherwise qualified services when the book is purchased. A well-versed specialist should be consulted if legal or technological guidance is needed.

The Declaration of Principles has been accepted and approved by a committee of the American Bar Association and a committee of Publishers and Associations. Any electronic or textual reproduction, repetition, or dissemination of any part of this document is forbidden. This publication's documentation and preservation are strictly prohibited, and preservation of this document is only allowed with the publisher's written permission. The rights to intellectual property are reserved.

The material provided herein is believed to be accurate and consistent, with the consumer bearing full responsibility for any liability resulting from the usage or violation of any laws, protocols, or instructions contained herein, whether due to inattention or otherwise.

In no condition will the publisher be found liable for any reparation, negligence, or monetary injury incurred as a result of the details contained herein, whether explicitly or indirectly. The copyrights not owned by the publisher belong to the writer.

The information presented here is solely for instructional purposes and is thus universal. The information is provided without some sort of guarantee or arrangement. The trademarks are used without the permission or backing of the trademark owner, and the trademark is written without the permission or backing of the trademark owner. The trademarks and labels listed in this book are the property of their respective owners, and this text is not associated with them.

Table of contents

<u>Introduction</u>

Emotional eating may be soothing in the short term, but in this book we expose why it's not the healthiest choice in the long run. If you're an emotional eater, you might eat to relieve tension and depression, increase pleasure, and provide warmth. Overeating, on the other side, adds to weight gain, heart failure, asthma, and a slew of other health concerns. Here are some Myths and Realities about emotional eating that should make you rethink how you deal with life's stressors, disappointments, and other feelings.

Overeating isn't uncommon — just think about Thanksgiving, as you stuff yourself silly. Although there's a major gap between occasional overeating and binge eating disorder, which is a psychiatric disease (BED). Binge eating is associated with feelings of depression, shame, and powerlessness. It's not about partying — that's probably one of the many stereotypes about this illness. Here we will discuss the strategies and some coping techniques that will help you to be emotionally independent.

Emotional eating isn't about meeting the body's basic nutritional requirements for energy. It's about saturating the blood with carbohydrates on a regular basis, as a result of a loss of emotional discipline, a profound psychiatric illness that must be bravely confronted and medically monitored.

While diets have existed since Adam and Eve had to reduce their dessert choices, it wasn't until the 1960's that our collective consciousness around weight loss moved into high gear. It expanded to our current degree of fascination within a few decades. We consume more food-related content and have more representations of food in the media and climate than the majority of the world's population. This relentless emphasis on diet and weight will only help to enhance the latent urge to overeat.

It is important that we learn to manage tension in our daily lives. Emotional eating can't be completely eliminated and it's a function of everyday life. We should, however, learn to relieve stress, anxiety using strategies like exercise, mindfulness, yoga, time management, and support programs, giving us more power over our already set eating behaviors and their impacts on our physical and mental well-being.

Chapter 1. Emotional Eating - Causes and Facts

Emotional eating is the urge of sufferers to feed in response to unpleasant or difficult thoughts, particularly though they are not physically hungry. Mental eating, also known as emotional appetite, is characterized by a need for high-calorie or high-carbohydrate items with little nutritional benefit. Comfort snacks, such as ice cream, cakes, chocolate, popcorn, French fries, and pizza, are often craved by emotional eaters. When anxious, about 40% of people eat more, 40% eat less, and 20% eat the same volume. As a result, depression is linked to both weight gain and weight loss.

Although emotional eating may be a sign of atypical depression, often individuals who do not have psychiatric depression or any other mental health disorder partake in this behavior in reaction to fleeting emotions or long-term stress. This is a very normal condition that is critical because it may make it impossible to follow a healthier diet and lead to obesity.

Is It Really That Depression Makes You Fat?

The Stress Hormone Cortisol

Since excess cortisol is secreted at periods of physical or psychological discomfort, and the usual cycle of cortisol secretion (with amounts greatest in the morning and lowest at night) may be disrupted, cortisol has been dubbed the "stress hormone." Cortisol secretion destruction can not only facilitate weight gain, but it may also influence where the weight is stored in the body. According to some research, depression and high cortisol levels affect fat accumulation in the abdomen region rather than the hips. Since abdominal fat deposition is closely connected to the occurrence of cardiovascular disease, including heart attacks and strokes, this fat deposition has been nicknamed "toxic fat."

When it comes to emotional eating and binge eating, what's the difference?

The volume of food eaten is the main distinction between emotional eating and binge eating. Although all include a feeling of difficulty suppressing a food craving, emotional eating can involve consuming small or large amounts of food and maybe the only sign of a mental condition such as obesity, bulimia, or binge eating disorder, or it may be a result of one. Binge eating disorder is a psychiatric condition marked by repeated periods of compulsive overeating in which affected individuals ingest a quantity of food that is far greater than what other people consume in a specific time frame (for example, over two hours) except though they are not hungry. An individual suffering from a binge eating disorder can eat far more quickly than normal, hide the amount they eat out of embarrassment and feel disgusted by their food afterward. The binges must occur on average once a week over three months to apply for this condition.

What are the causes, triggers, and risk factors?

Emotional eating, like other emotional signs, is considered to be the product of a combination of causes rather than a particular source. Girls and women are at a greater risk for eating disorders, according to some studies, and they are often at a higher risk for emotional eating. Another study shows that men are more likely to eat excessively in response to feeling stressed or upset, whereas women are more likely to eat excessively in response to failing a diet in certain communities.

The symptoms of a rise in the hormone cortisol, which is one of the body's reactions to stress, are believed to be close to those of the drug prednisone. Both appear to trigger the body's stress mechanism (fight or flight), which includes elevated pulse and respiratory rates, the blood supply to tissues, and visual acuity. Increased appetite is also a part of the stress reaction to provide the body with the strength it requires to combat or escape, resulting in cravings for so-called comfort foods. People that have been exposed to persistent stress (such as work, education, or family stress, or exposure to violence or abuse) are more likely to have excessively elevated cortisol levels in their bodies, which may lead to the development of chronic emotional-eating habits.

Emotional eating is a psychological condition in which people associate food with warmth, strength, good emotions, or some other cause other than supplying nutrition to their bodies. When they are physically complete, they can eat to fill an emotional void and indulge in mindless eating. Some people who eat their emotions may have been raised to associate food with feelings rather than sustenance, particularly if the food was limited or often used as a reward or punishment, or as a replacement for emotional intimacy.

What are the signs and symptoms of emotional eating?

A desire to become painfully hungry all of a time, rather than steadily as in a real physical urge to eat triggered by an empty stomach, is one of the warning signs of emotional eating. Emotional eaters are more likely to consume fast food than to seek out healthy meals, and the need to eat is normally accompanied by tension or an unpleasant feeling, such as depression, disappointment, rage, remorse, or annoyance. Other characteristics of emotional eating include a loss of control when eating and frequent regret over what has been consumed.

What types of Professionals deal with emotional eating?

When emotional eating leads to overweight or obesity, a variety of health care providers may assess and manage it, as well as assist in weight loss. Since this symptom can appear at any point during a person's existence, it can be addressed by anyone from pediatricians to family doctors to other primary care physicians. Emotional-eating patients can be cared for by clinicians, medical practitioners, and physician assistants. Psychiatrists, behavioral psychologists, social workers, and certified counselors are among the mental health providers who are often interested in identifying and addressing this issue. Although all of these professionals can assist patients who suffer from emotional eating, it's possible that more than one of them will collaborate to help the individual solve this symptom.

What approaches do physicians use to recognize emotional eating?

After confirming that the sufferer has undergone a clinical assessment and test work to ensure that the disorder is not part of a neurological or other medical illness like Prader-Willi syndrome, the diagnosis of emotional eating is created. The patient might be asked a set of questions from a structured questionnaire or self-test as part of the behavioral wellbeing portion of the assessment to better determine the presence of emotional eating. Emotional eating can be differentiated from such eating conditions such as bulimia, binge eating, or pica by a thorough examination of the background of mental health symptoms. A mental well-being specialist will likely look to see whether there are any other mental disorders involved.

<u>Chapter: 2. Myths That are True</u>

Comfort foods are distinct for men and women

There is a differentiation between men and women. Men prefer soft, hearty, meal-related comfort foods (think roast, casseroles, and soup), while women prefer snack foods, according to research (think chocolate and ice cream).

Feeling guilty for eating cake has a negative impact on weight reduction

Eating cake while feeling guilty leads to a slower weight loss. The cake is comfort food that is often linked to feelings of regret and worry, as well as satisfaction and relaxation. Dieters who correlated cake with "guilt" rather than "celebration" were less likely to lose weight in one report. Dieters who experienced happy emotions, such as joy and warmth from the cake, were more likely to lose weight. Guilt has the power to derail your efforts.

We crave familiar comfort foods

We consume comfort foods because it's what we've always done. When we're nervous, we return to the things we consume most, whether they're safe or not. Students were more inclined to select the snacks they consume more often at high tension periods, according to researchers who followed their eating patterns among college students during midterm exams. Choosing common foods needs less thinking and commitment.

Ritual provides a sense of security

Ritual provides a sense of security and pleasure. Will you have a favorite way to consume comfort foods? Do you really take the icing off the cupcake first, or do you always split the peanut butter sandwich in half? Food is consumed in a variety of forms by most of us. And the positive emotions we get from these little routines are backed up by science. Eaters who created a custom out of unwrapping and progressively splitting bits of a chocolate bar not only felt the pleasant relaxation emotions, but they also liked the chocolate better than those who just unwrapped and consumed the chocolate, according to a report reported in the journal Psychological Research.

Feeding is an act of emotion

It's not all about the flavor. We also assume that comfort foods taste good whether they taste good or that consuming them feels good. In a study published in the Journal of Clinical Investigation, researchers were able to evoke the same emotions and memories by inserting a fat-based substance directly into the stomachs of the subjects. The researchers then caused depression in the participants and discovered that those who obtained the fat-based solution had a lower brain reaction to sadness on MRI tests than those who received the dummy or placebo solution. Many that were given the "comfort" cure didn't have that much pain. This prompted the researchers to believe that something hormonal is activated in the gut, and then sends messages to the brain, making us feel healthy.

Happy people overeat too

Emotional eating is triggered by both positive and negative emotions. According to the journal, sometimes positive thoughts cause cravings for comfort foods. In reality, positive people are more prone to overeat than sad people, which is a little-known fact.

Chicken soup is a perfect company

Chicken soup is soothing and will help you feel less lonely. This is why: People who consumed chicken noodle soup were less sad when consuming it, according to a report reported in Psychological Research. They were also able to come up with more relational terms to explain their emotions while eating it. To put it another way, if you consume the soup when chatting to others, you're more likely to speak with them. Comfort meals equal soothing emotions, which equals comfort in the company of others.

We always need comfort food

At the end of the day, comfort is sought. Take a peek at some of the more popular "last meals" requested by death row inmates: Fried foods were chosen by 67 percent, and desserts by 66 percent. Is it so surprising that they crave calorie-dense comfort foods?

While you're away from family, familiar foods are comforting

Eating common comfort foods, according to a survey of students studying abroad in England, offered emotional help and provided a "taste of home" comfort. If you live abroad for a long time, experts warn that you'll start to miss the fresh foods in your acculturated diet in the same way you craved your native land's comfort foods.

Dieters are the ones that are more vulnerable to comfort food

Dieters are the people that are more likely to feed mentally. People who are at risk for emotional eating under stress, according to experts, have a high BMI, express "low" or "moody" emotions, and have a high cortisol reactivity (your body's response to stress). However, studies have shown that attempting to step back and exercise discipline usually backfires!

The level of comfort is dose-dependent

That's right! When emotional eaters were offered a small amount of chocolate (about one-ninth of a

Hershey's bar), there were no shifts of attitude. Unfortunately, it took a lot of chocolate to even create a dent in attitude, and as we have learned, it's just a temporary "feel nice" practice!

Chapter 3. Myths that are False

Myth #1: Emotional eating is not the same as all types of eating

Eating is an intense experience. Attempts to exclude emotion from eating improve the implicit motivation to consume foods with higher emotional and sensory quality (taste, smell, texture, sweet, salty, fat). That's why broccoli is never a good substitute for chocolate.

Attempts to eliminate emotion from eating lead to "deprivation motivations," an urge to get as many as possible because supplies last when availability is restricted or prohibited. Note that only one tiny slice of fruit was prohibited to Adam and Eve; equate that to the list of items we're not supposed to consume on diets.

Since we can't take the emotion out of food, long-term weight loss is based on which emotions drive us. The choice is to choose between core pain and core worth.

Disregard, insignificance, shame, devaluation, disrespect, rejection, powerlessness, inadequacy, or unlovability are all feeling the core hurt eating seeks to stop. It's impossible to ignore the connection between core pain and high-energy, high-sensory food. For a few minutes, fast feeding of high sensory, high-calorie food numbs pain and restores vitality; for a few minutes, rapid eating of high sensory, high-calorie food numbs pain and restores energy.

Quick eating causes core pain. We realize that if we stop, our core pains will worsen and our vitality will disappear. As a result, we don't rest unless our bodies tell us to. Overeating becomes "attacks on food" when central hurts are serious and the ability to control them is underdeveloped, rendering food harmful rather than nourishing, an instrument of damage rather than a source of well-being and well-being.

Eating is a type of self-expression. Rather than dwelling on what you don't have, you reflect on increasing the meaning of your life. It encourages you to move your attention away from weight and diet and toward love toward yourself and others. When you place a higher priority on yourself, you will naturally place a higher value on your fitness and well-being, and you will learn to inspire yourself by "acts of kindness."

Myth #2: If I lose weight, I would have a higher self-esteem

Weight loss plans emphasize this message both clearly and implicitly by emphasizing "goals" and "orders," as in "Think of how you don't like looking in the mirror."

"You should embrace yourself overweight," they might suggest, or "Keep walking, even though you relapse." Yet no amount of lip service will substitute for the mental effects of goals: if you don't meet them, you're a loser.

Over-eaters already sound like failures when it comes to weight management. But, just in case it wasn't enough to guarantee defeat, weight reduction plans' targets and rules have a built-in failure mechanism, simply because all winners are also losers. We sacrifice as much as we gain in something that lasts a long period, such as a lifelong motivation to feed. It's just regression to the mean; once you collect enough data, such as test scores, the mean result, or average score, becomes more common when anomalies from the mean become less so.

If you "gain" by hitting your weight reduction target, figures suggest that you would most definitely "lose" by relapsing at some stage in your life (hopefully earlier rather than later). "I dropped 200 pounds this year, but I added 210," goes the old joke. Goals and guidelines around food are more apt to elicit core hurts (guilty and insufficient) than core values, setting you up for failure.

The weakest aspect of this misconception — that you would love yourself more if you lose weight — is that it distorts a plain truth: You will not lose weight until you value yourself more.

Is it the loved self or the devalued self that is more prone to binge eat and attack food (or to be a bad partner or abuser, for that matter)?

Myth #3: We eat so much when we're bored

Boredom's innate motivation is to pursue something interesting to do. You don't eat to escape boredom; instead, you get involved in something. Boredom just encourages people to overeat as it threatens their heart hurts. When boredom makes me feel unimportant or insufficient, my subconscious misinterprets the decline in energy and well-being as hunger, raising my odds of overeating.

Myth #4: We eat to feel better

Many publications have encouraged us to create lists of our "favorite foods," which include items like pizza, oatmeal, cookies, chicken and dumplings, ice cream, and so on. The manufacturers of alcohol and Valium would be out of business if these foods provided substantial comforting qualities.

It has little to do with the food and more to do with their core principle, why certain people feel comforted after consuming those foods. They get the impression that they are "taking care of themselves," because they should not overeat. When a central principle motivates food (or something else), relaxation and overall well-being are possible outcomes.

However, if core hurts drive "comfort food," the outcome would be remorse and shame. When you think about it, it's a little silly to suggest you consume for pleasure when overeating creates serious physical and emotional pain.

Myth #5: We eat because we enjoy it (because our mothers expressed affection with food).

This is a particularly harmful myth. Over-eaters of missing mothers are advised that they eat for attention because their mothers did not show devotion for food from the very individuals who support it. Ok, guess what? Food is a fairly popular way to show love. In general, most mothers use food to show love to their children, even those who grow up to be thin; nevertheless, parents who make a huge deal of the type of food their children consume are more likely to have eating disorders.

Aside from empirical evidence, "eating for love," like "eating for warmth," defies logic. Overeating contributes to self-loathing and resentment, but not to affection. Is anybody ever experienced love as a result of overeating? If we did, we'd savor it, prolong it, and stretch it out as far as possible. Overeaters, particularly those who attack food, have a tendency to eat at a single speed: quick and furious. Some people will binge until they are completely satisfied, only to feel so terrible for themselves that they will finally adhere to their weight reduction targets. Self-loathing, on the other hand, just encourages you to engage in self-destructive acts.

Since core hurt eating is not an effort to feel appreciated, welcomed, or cherished, we don't eat for affection. Core wounds, on the other hand, are about feeling incapable of worth, recognition, and affection. A feeling of unworthiness triggers a significant drop in well-being and energy, which strengthens the need to feed.

Eating is a pleasurable experience

True, but it's just for three minutes. Research published in the Journal of Appetite looked into how long chocolate makes you feel healthy. Comfort and bliss, it turned out, just last 3 minutes. Three minutes! Isn't it amazing how brief comfort food can be?

Everybody suffers from the same hunger pangs

Comfort items aren't universal. Do you think chocolate is the world's favorite feel-good food? It's not the case. People in various countries seek relief from various foods. Miso soup, okay (rice porridge served to sick children), and ramen are common comfort foods in Japan. Samosas, potato-stuffed crisps served with spicy green chutney, are a common snack in India. It's new pasta or potato gnocchi in Italy.

Hormones are responsible for chocolate cravings

Hormonal chocolate cravings are not triggered by PMS. You may believe that the hormones cause you to desire chocolate at the time of the month, but despite no longer getting periods, 80 percent of menopausal women experience chocolate cravings. Experts agree that our need for warmth, coupled with our anxiety regarding our cycle, drives us to use a culturally reinforced coping mechanism. To put it another way, we expect chocolate to benefit, so we continue to desire it, rather than hormones leading us to it.

When it comes to comfort meals, money is irrelevant

Among those on public assistance, Kraft macaroni isn't much of a comfort. The famous Kraft macaroni and cheese dinner is often listed as a comfort meal among middle-income people who do not struggle to pay for food. For some who aren't sure how they'll budget for their next meal, though, it's just the same. Since this cheesy packaged lunch is often given to food banks, it runs the risk of being a monotonous staple for recipients, reinforcing their loss of financial strength and meal options.

<u>Chapter 4. Solutions of Emotional Eating</u>

4.1. Useful Suggestions

- A few useful suggestions should be implemented while we are feeling both up and down in times of celebration, joy, or down while we might be feeling down or nervous in an attempt to disrupt this loop of possible addiction or emotional intake of food, and they include the following.

- Maintaining a food diary about what you consume, how much you eat, how hungry you are, and how you feel during the day will help you find causes.

- Reducing discomfort that could be leading to overeating or reward eating by going on a stroll, breathing exercises, yoga, or engaging in a favorite hobby.

- Do a hunger fact check to determine if you are experiencing physical or mental hunger.

- Seek assistance from relatives, friends, or treatment staff.

- Combat boredom by contacting a mate, heading for a stroll, playing a game, listening to music, or reading to prevent the mind from drifting to food-related thinking.

- Remove the lure by making your home and office a secure refuge free of things that are commonly borrowed for convenience.

- Don't deny yourself of anything. We cannot deny ourselves fundamental needs like food, unlike those recovering from opioid abuse or alcoholism who would abstain from such drugs. Cravings may be exacerbated by putting too many restrictions on yourself or eating the same ingredients over and over. To bring diversity to your diet, consume a satisfying amount of nutritious foods and indulge in a treat every now and then.

- Snack on fruits, vegetables, nuts, and un-buttered popcorn for a nutritious snack.

- Learn from your mistakes: Whenever you have an emotional eating crisis, forgive yourself and try again with your next meal. Do not write off the day or yourself as a total disappointment. We are just human, and life happens. We will always fall into these traps, and how we survive and evolve will determine our success. Learn from the experience and make constructive changes to avoid such occurrences in the future.

4.2.　What is the right way to cope with emotional eating?

Overcoming emotional eating typically involves educating the sufferer healthy ways to perceive food and cultivate improved eating behaviors, as well as identifying their reasons for participating in this behavior and improving effective stress prevention and coping strategies.

1. Exercise is an effective part of stress management since it reduces the release of stress hormones, which may contribute to a reduction of depression, anxiety, and insomnia, as well as a decline in the propensity to partake in emotional eating.

2. Meditation and other calming strategies are both efficient methods to relieve depression and, as a result, minimize emotional eating. As a consequence, performing one to two mediation exercises per day may have long-term health advantages, including reducing elevated blood pressure and heart rate.

3. Other effective strategies to effectively alleviate stress include abstaining from opioid usage and drinking no more than small levels of alcohol since both of these drugs heighten the body's reaction to stress. Indulging in the usage of such drugs often prohibits the individual from confronting

their issues head-on, preventing them from developing successful coping or stress-reduction strategies.

4. Such stress-reducing lifestyle improvements include having breaks at home and at college. Avoid cramming so much into your schedule. Recognize the stressors and react appropriately. Take daily vacation days at times that are comfortable for you. Structure your life so that you can adapt to the unpredictable in a relaxed manner.

5. Psychotropic drugs, especially selective serotonin reuptake inhibitors (SSRIs), may be incredibly effective if stress triggers a full-blown psychological condition such as posttraumatic stress disorder (PTSD), clinical depression, or anxiety disorders. Sertraline (Zoloft), paroxetine (Paxil), fluoxetine (Prozac), citalopram (Celexa), and escitalopram are examples of SSRIs (Lexapro).

4.3. What are the chances of emotional eating if left untreated?

Emotional overeating, if left unchecked, will contribute to problems such as difficulty losing weight, obesity, and even the initiation of food addiction. People who are vulnerable to emotional eating, on the other hand, are also more open to stress mitigation in correcting their propensity to emotionally eat than people who eat less while stressed.

4.4.   Is there a way to avoid emotional eating?

Reduced discomfort, healthy approaches to consider and control feelings, and treating food as sustenance rather than a means to fix issues are also essential factors in avoiding emotional eating (eating to live rather than living to eat). Emotional eating is often prevented by dreaming about the potential rather than focusing on meeting food cravings, according to research. Meditation, yoga, and other positive tension prevention and stress management strategies, as well as limiting caffeine, alcohol, and medications, are also good approaches to avoid unhealthy eating habits.

Conclusion

The blunt truth to this issue is that it does happen, and it is not restricted to women. It is important to have a safe or positive relationship with food. Many of what we do as a group revolves around the idea of using food to commemorate both happy and sad events of our lives. Comfort foods like fried chicken, burgers, and casseroles are high in fat; high sweet products like sweets, desserts, and pies are high in sugar; and high starch items like bread, rice, and pasta are high in carbohydrate. We seldom pause to consider how these events would affect us at the moment. Its aim is to fill a hole. Our ingestion of these foods will trigger our brain's instant reward receptors, making us feel happier and need more. A person or community stress-management treatment may be really beneficial for those who require assistance coping with stress. Stress counseling and community therapy have been found to enhance mental well-being and reduce stress symptoms.

This insatiable need or drive is similar to an addiction, and it exists regardless of our appetite. These habits can lead to an unbalanced diet, which can accelerate the development of obesity. The bidirectional relationship between our mood and obesity becomes entangled, allowing each disease state to feed off the other. It's likely that you'll feel sad or nervous as a consequence of your weight. The framework of "When I'm down, I eat to feel stronger" on the other side, may become a constant feedback loop and cycle that causes an individual to suffer. This book will provide you a real insight into the Myths and Realities of Emotional Eating and comprehensive coping-strategies to fight your fears and to become emotionally independent well-being.